Olivia and the Dummy Fairy

No More Binkies

By Andrea Locket

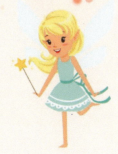

OLIVIA LOVED HER DUMMY SHE HAD IT WITH HER ALL THE TIME.

SHE EVEN HAD IT WHEN SHE GOT HER TOY BOX OUT TO PLAY WITH HER BEAR AND STACKING BRICKS.

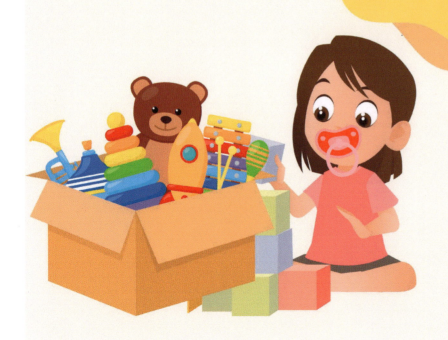

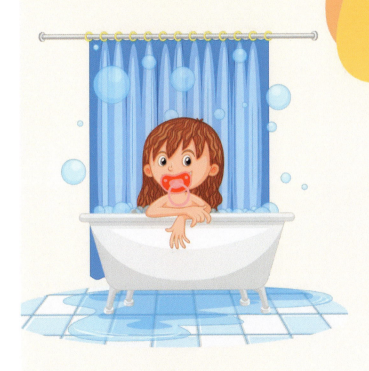

Dummy went with her everywhere.

She'd not even take it out when she had a bath!

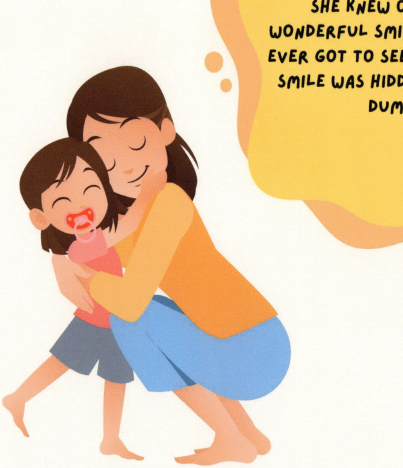

IT WAS MAKING MOM A LITTLE SAD. SHE KNEW OLIVA HAD A WONDERFUL SMILE, BUT NOBODY EVER GOT TO SEE IT. HER LOVELY SMILE WAS HIDDEN BEHIND HER DUMMY.

MOM TRIED TO PERSUADE OLIVIA TO GIVE UP HER DUMMY. BUT IT DIDN'T WORK. OLIVIA HAD DUMMIES HIDDEN ALL OVER THE HOUSE.

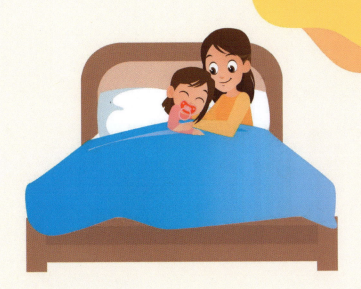

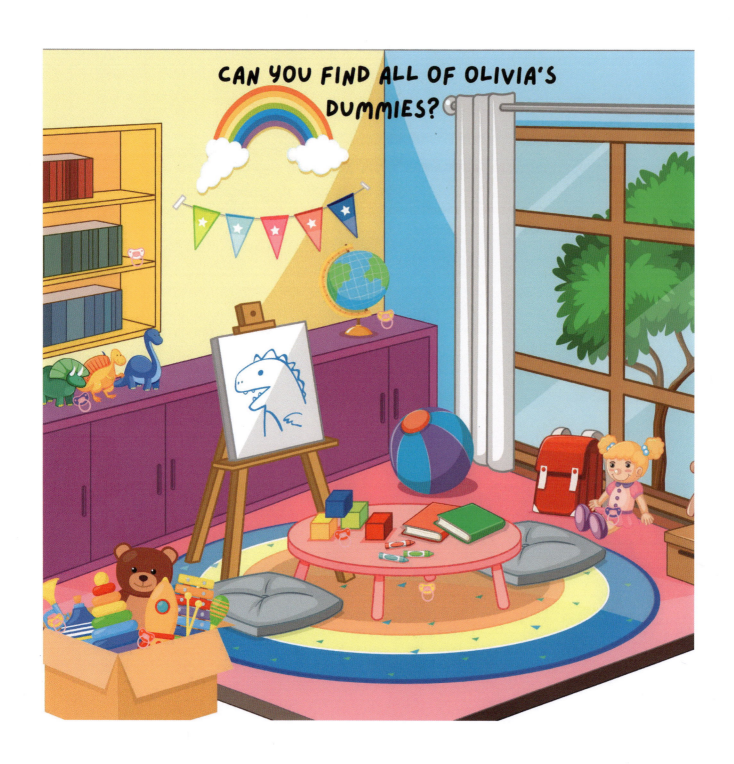

DID YOU FIND THEM ALL?

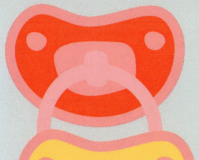 THERE WERE TWO RED ONES

THREE YELLOW ONES

TWO BLUE ONES

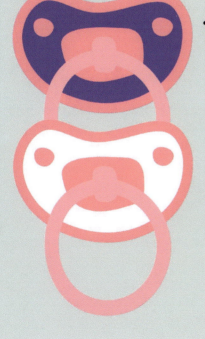 AND ONE WHITE ONE

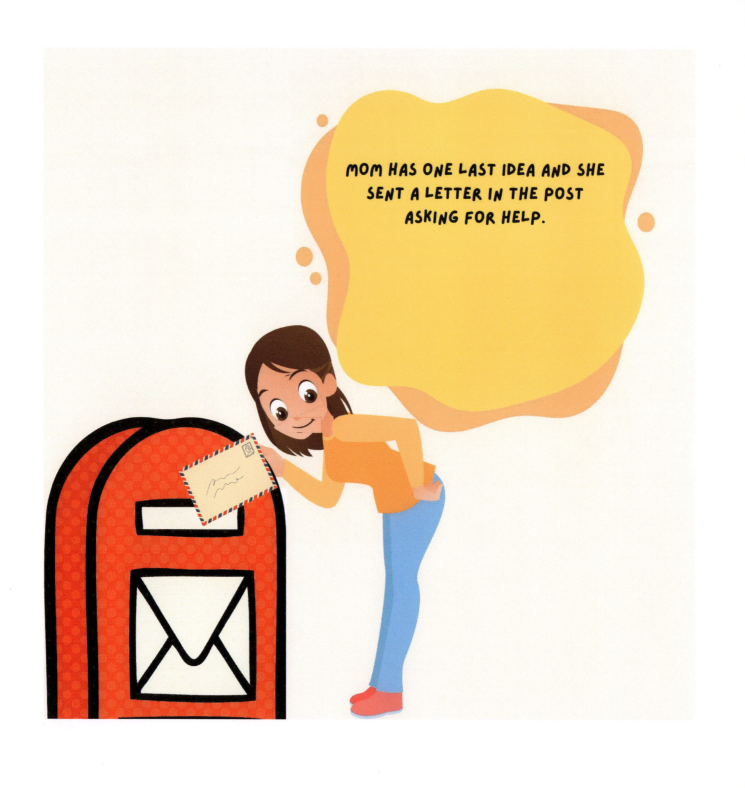

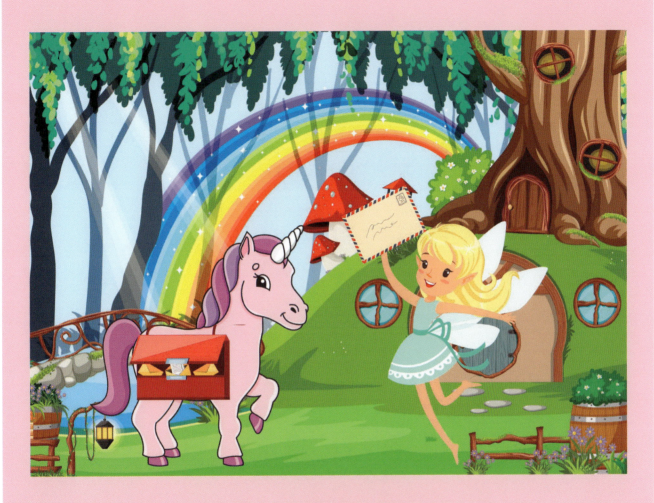

MOM'S LETTER ARRIVES IN FAIRYLAND

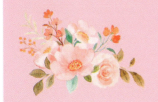

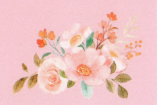

Mom's letter makes it all the way to fairyland.

Emily the unicorn delivers it to Sophie the dummy fairy.

Sophie is the best dummy fairy there has ever been

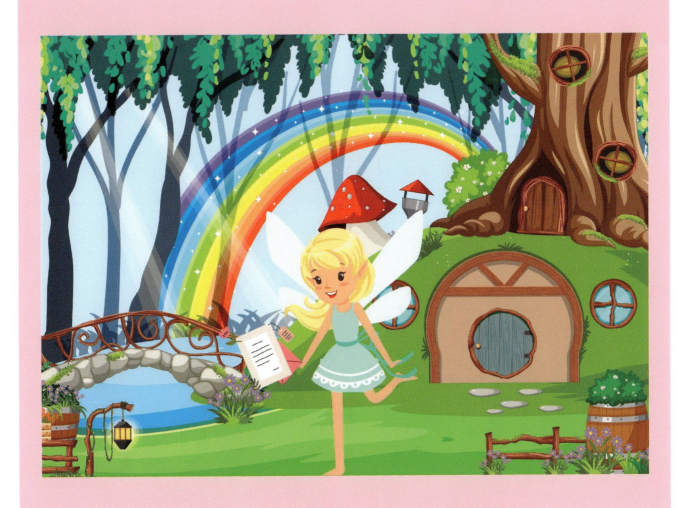

SOPHIE READS MOM'S LETTER

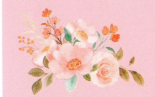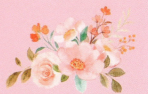

SOPHIE LAUGHS WHEN SHE READS THE LETTER. SHE CAN REMEMBER OLIVIA'S MOM. ONE OF THE TOUGHEST CASES SHE'D EVER HAD. OLIVIA'S MOM HADN'T WANTED TO GIVE UP HER DUMMY WHEN SHE WAS LITTLE.
SOPHIE SETS OFF TO VISIT OLIVIA.

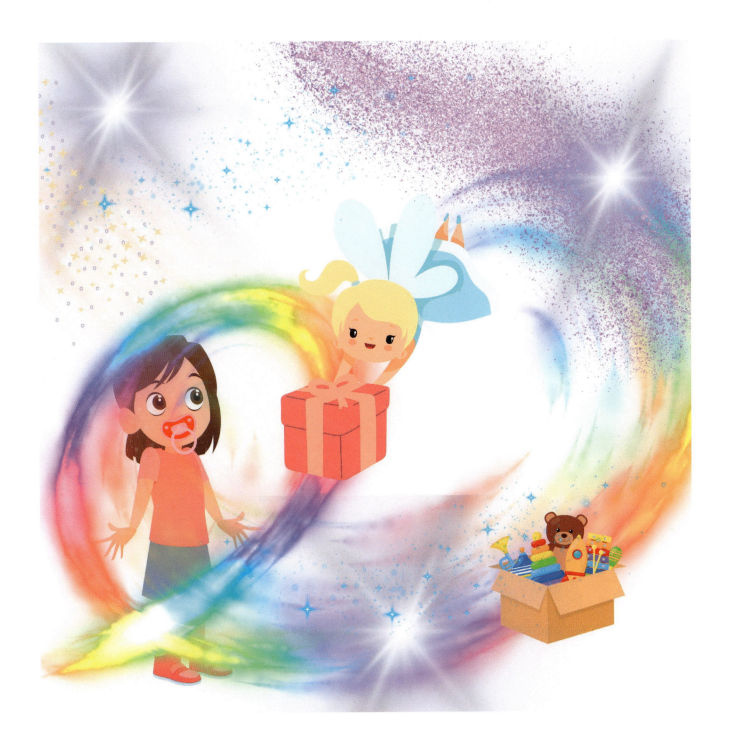

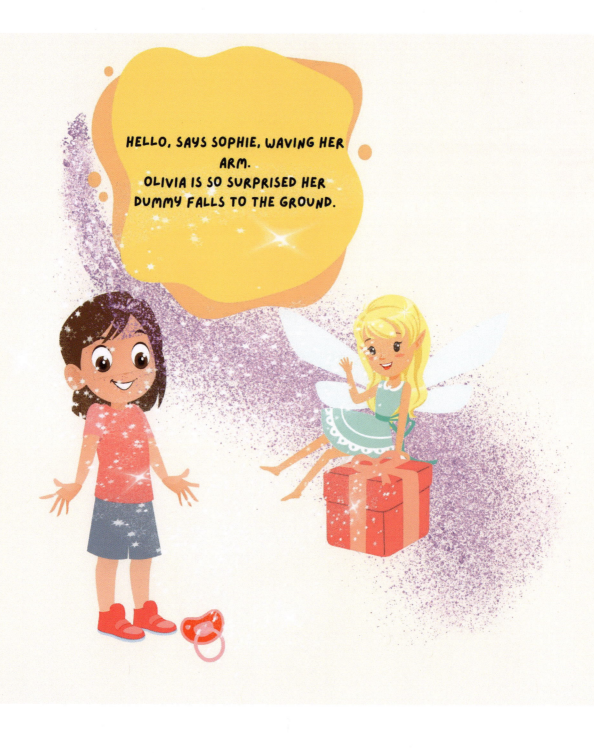

All around Olivia there are glittering stars and puffs of magic dust.

"Your mom wrote me a letter and asked me to call. She wanted me to release your smile," says Sophie.

"I don't understand,' says Olivia. "I've not lost my smile and it's not trapped anywhere?"

Sophie laughs, and whispers, "You need to stop hiding your bright smile behind a dummy."

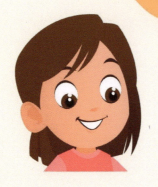
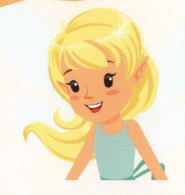

"IT'S TRAPPED BEHIND A DUMMY AND WE CAN'T SEE WHETHER YOU ARE HAPPY OR SAD," SOPHIE EXPLAINED. "AND THE DREAM FAIRY WON'T KNOW WHAT SORT OF DREAMS TO BRING YOU IF SHE CAN'T SEE YOUR SMILE."

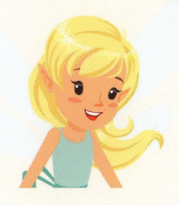

"I DIDN'T KNOW THAT," SAID OLIVIA. "BUT I DON'T WANT TO GIVE MY DUMMY UP, I LIKE IT. I ALWAYS HAVE IT."

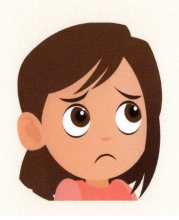
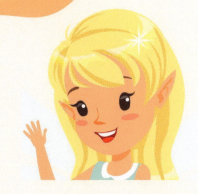

"ARE YOU SURE YOU NEED IT?" SOPHIE SAYS. "WHEN I ARRIVED IT FELL OUT OF YOUR MOUTH AND YOU'VE NOT EVEN LOOKED FOR IT."

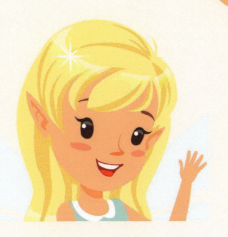

"WOW! YOU ARE RIGHT. I HADN'T NOTICED IT WAS MISSING AT ALL," SAID OLIVIA.

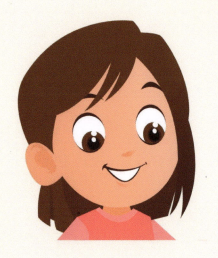

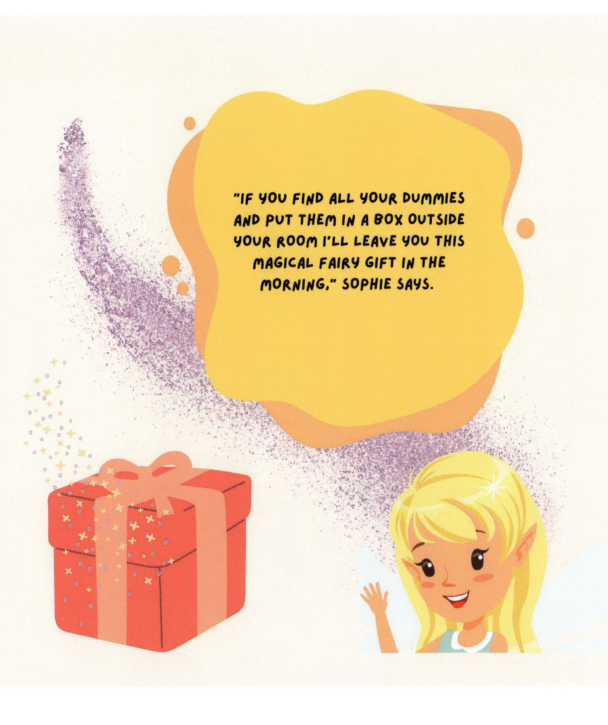

"IF YOU FIND ALL YOUR DUMMIES AND PUT THEM IN A BOX OUTSIDE YOUR ROOM I'LL LEAVE YOU THIS MAGICAL FAIRY GIFT IN THE MORNING," SOPHIE SAYS.

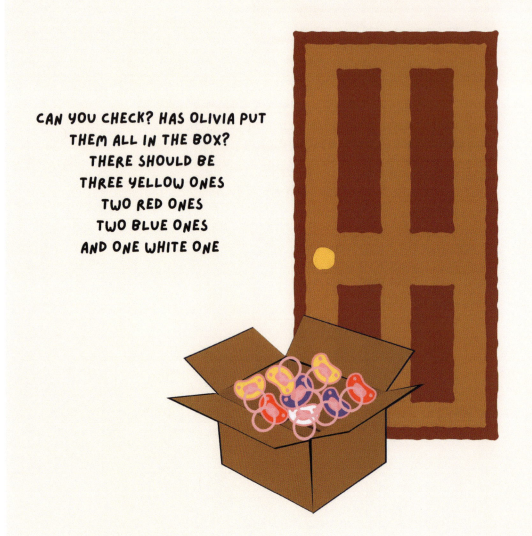

CAN YOU CHECK? HAS OLIVIA PUT
THEM ALL IN THE BOX?
THERE SHOULD BE
THREE YELLOW ONES
TWO RED ONES
TWO BLUE ONES
AND ONE WHITE ONE

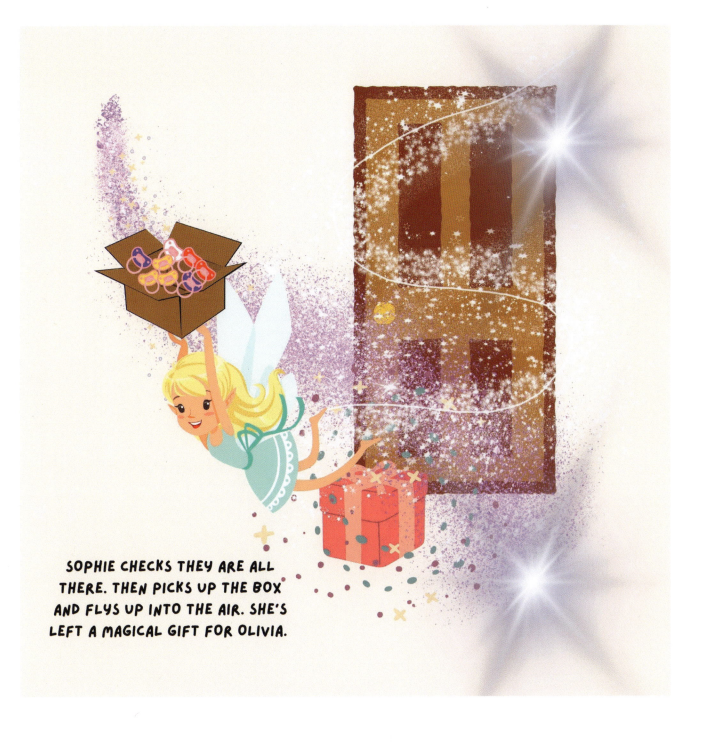

SOPHIE CHECKS THEY ARE ALL THERE. THEN PICKS UP THE BOX AND FLYS UP INTO THE AIR. SHE'S LEFT A MAGICAL GIFT FOR OLIVIA.

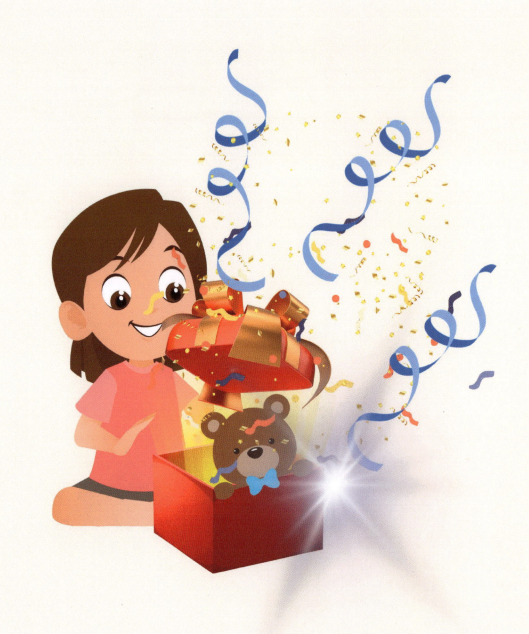

INSIDE IS A MAGICAL TEDDY FOR OLIVIA. SHE CAN HUG TEDDY ALL NIGHT AND HE'LL MAKE SURE SHE NEVER THINKS ABOUT HER DUMMY AGAIN.

WHY DON'T YOU GATHER UP ALL YOUR DUMMIES AND POP THEM IN A BOX OUTSIDE YOUR BEDROOM DOOR? SOPHIE THE DUMMY FAIRY MIGHT LEAVE YOU A LITTLE GIFT AS WELL.

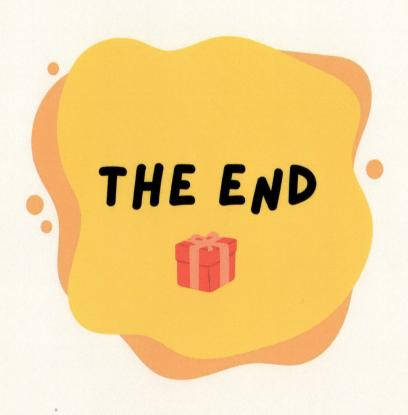

Printed in Great Britain
by Amazon

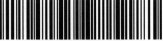